Gout Relief

Understanding its Triggers

In-Depth Exploration of Causes, Symptoms, Effective Management Strategies, Lifestyle Changes and Prevention

Graham Julian Oliver

Disclaimer

The information provided in this book is for educational and informational purposes only and is not intended as medical advice. The content is based on research and the author's personal experience and opinions. Readers are encouraged to consult with a qualified healthcare professional before making any decisions related to their health, especially concerning the prevention, management, and treatment of gout or any other medical condition.

The author and publisher do not warrant the completeness or accuracy of the information presented and shall not be liable for any damages arising from the use or inability to use this book. Individual results may vary, and the information provided may not be suitable for every reader. Any references made are solely for informational purposes, and readers are encouraged to do their own research and exercise caution when considering any products, services, or websites discussed. By reading this book, you acknowledge and agree to the terms of this disclaimer.

About This Book

The book titled "Gout Relief: Understanding its Triggers" serves as a comprehensive guide for individuals seeking to understand and manage this challenging form of arthritis. Gout is defined as a type of arthritis caused by the accumulation of uric acid crystals in the joints, leading to intense pain and inflammation. Recognizing the importance of understanding triggers for effective management is pivotal for those who experience gout, as it empowers them to identify and avoid factors that could lead to painful flare-ups. The book provides an overview of the common symptoms associated with gout attacks, including sudden joint pain, redness, swelling, and the potential for chronic issues such as tophi, or uric acid deposits. Additionally, it introduces lifestyle changes that can significantly aid in the prevention of future attacks, underscoring the need for a proactive approach to health.

Understanding the specific triggers of gout is essential for effective management. The book highlights that identifying personal triggers can not only help prevent painful attacks but also foster a deeper awareness of dietary and lifestyle factors that contribute to the condition. It emphasizes the importance of consulting healthcare professionals to gain a comprehensive understanding of how gout interacts with overall health. By exploring these triggers, readers are equipped with the knowledge to take control of their health and make informed decisions about their diet and lifestyle.

The text delves into the causes of gout, including hyperuricemia or high uric acid levels, which play a central role in the development of this condition. It discusses genetic predisposition, dietary influences, and the impact of dehydration, as well as medical conditions like hypertension that can trigger gout. Lifestyle factors, such as alcohol consumption and obesity, are also examined in detail. The book provides a thorough overview of how hormonal factors and age contribute to gout occurrences, alongside the less commonly recognized triggers, such as stress and high-fructose corn syrup. Understanding these diverse causes equips readers with a well-rounded perspective on managing and preventing gout.

The symptoms of gout are vividly described, outlining the sudden onset of joint pain and the accompanying signs of inflammation. Readers will gain insight into the typical affected joints, with a particular focus on the big toe, and learn to differentiate acute flare-ups from chronic symptoms. This understanding is crucial for early recognition and intervention, allowing individuals to seek appropriate medical care in a timely manner.

The book emphasizes the importance of a thorough diagnosis, detailing the role of medical history, physical examinations, and various diagnostic tests, including joint aspiration and blood tests to measure uric acid levels. By understanding the diagnostic process, readers can better navigate their healthcare journey and ensure they receive accurate and effective treatment.

Effective management strategies are central to this guide, including the use of medications like NSAIDs and corticosteroids during flare-ups, as well as the introduction of urate-lowering therapy (ULT). Lifestyle modifications are equally crucial, with a strong emphasis on maintaining hydration, making dietary adjustments, and incorporating regular exercise into daily routines. The book encourages individuals to develop personalized gout management plans and emphasizes the significance of ongoing monitoring of uric acid levels.

Dietary considerations are explored in depth, providing readers with essential knowledge about foods high in purines that should be avoided and suggesting low-purine alternatives. This section highlights the importance of a balanced diet for overall health and emphasizes the role of hydration, dairy products, and whole grains in reducing gout risk. The text also addresses the impact of sugar-sweetened beverages and processed foods, making it clear how dietary choices can significantly influence gout management.

Preventing gout flare-ups necessitates meaningful lifestyle changes, and the book outlines various strategies for maintaining a healthy weight, managing stress, and establishing a regular exercise routine. The importance of hydration and the need for smoking cessation are underscored, alongside tips for incorporating mindfulness into daily life. Setting achievable health goals and tracking progress through journaling are presented as effective methods for fostering long-term change.

Alternative therapies offer additional avenues for relief, with discussions on herbal remedies, acupuncture, and homeopathy. The book encourages open dialogue with healthcare providers regarding the use of alternative treatments, emphasizing the importance of evidence-based practices in managing gout. Techniques like hot and cold therapy, dietary supplements, and engaging in gentle activities such as tai chi are explored as complementary options for pain relief and stress management.

Monitoring and follow-up care are critical components of managing gout, and the book stresses the significance of regular check-ups, keeping a symptom diary, and understanding laboratory tests related to gout management. Open communication with healthcare providers and involving family members in care strategies are encouraged to ensure a holistic approach to treatment.

Finally, the book addresses common concerns and frequently asked questions about gout, offering clarity on issues such as joint involvement, long-term effects, dietary control, and the interplay between gout and other health conditions. By providing comprehensive and practical information, "Gout Relief: Understanding its Triggers" serves as an invaluable resource for anyone seeking to take control of their gout journey through informed choices and proactive management.

Table of Contents

Introduction:

Definition of Gout as a Form of Arthritis

Gout is a type of arthritis characterized by sudden, severe pain, swelling, and redness in the affected joints, most commonly the big toe. It results from the body's inability to properly eliminate uric acid, leading to elevated levels that can crystallize in joints and surrounding tissues, causing intense inflammation and discomfort.

Understanding gout is essential for those affected, as it not only impacts daily life but can also lead to chronic joint damage if left unmanaged. By recognizing it as a chronic condition requiring attention, individuals can take proactive steps to reduce the frequency and severity of attacks.

Explanation of Uric Acid Crystals Forming in Joints

Uric acid is a waste product produced when the body breaks down purines, substances found in various foods and drinks. When the kidneys cannot filter out enough uric acid, or when the body produces too much, it can accumulate in the blood and form sharp crystals in the joints, leading to painful gout attacks.

To prevent the formation of these crystals, individuals should aim to manage uric acid levels through dietary choices and hydration. Staying well-hydrated helps dilute uric acid in the bloodstream, making it less likely to crystallize in the joints.

Importance of Understanding Triggers for Effective Management

Identifying and understanding gout triggers is crucial for effective management and prevention of flare-ups. Common triggers include certain foods high in purines, such as red meats, shellfish, and alcoholic beverages, especially beer. Stress and dehydration can also increase the likelihood of a gout attack.

To effectively manage gout, individuals should keep a journal to track their diet and symptoms. This practice can help pinpoint specific foods or activities that contribute to flare-ups, allowing for more informed lifestyle adjustments and better control over the condition.

Overview of Common Symptoms Experienced During a Gout Attack

A gout attack often begins suddenly, typically at night, presenting as intense pain in the affected joint, with the big toe being the most common site. Other symptoms may include redness, swelling, and warmth in the area, with the pain often described as excruciating and limiting mobility.

Recognizing these symptoms early can prompt individuals to seek timely treatment, such as taking anti-inflammatory medications or applying ice to the affected joint. Prompt action can significantly alleviate pain and reduce the duration of the flare-up.

Brief Introduction to the Lifestyle Changes That Can Help Prevent Gout Flare-Ups

Making specific lifestyle changes can play a significant role in preventing gout flare-ups. Key strategies include maintaining a healthy weight, staying hydrated, and consuming a balanced diet low in purines. Foods rich in whole grains, fruits, and vegetables are beneficial, while limiting intake of red meat and sugary beverages is advisable.

Additionally, incorporating regular physical activity can help manage weight and improve overall health, thereby lowering the risk of gout attacks. Simple activities like walking, swimming, or cycling can be effective, along with avoiding sudden, intense exercise that may strain joints.

Why Understanding Triggers is Essential

Identifying Personal Triggers Can Lead to Better Management

To effectively manage gout, it's essential to identify your personal triggers. Common triggers include high-purine foods such as red meat, shellfish, and sugary beverages. Start a food diary to track your meals and any subsequent gout flare-ups. Note any patterns that emerge, helping you pinpoint specific foods or habits that provoke your symptoms.

- By recognizing your triggers, you can adjust your diet and lifestyle accordingly. For example, if you find that consuming beer exacerbates your symptoms, consider limiting or eliminating it from your diet. Additionally, staying hydrated by drinking plenty of water can help flush uric acid from your system and may reduce the likelihood of future attacks.

Awareness Helps Prevent Painful Gout Attacks

Being aware of the factors that contribute to gout can significantly reduce the frequency of painful attacks. Keep a list of your known triggers and consult it regularly, especially when planning meals or social activities. This proactive approach can help you make informed choices that minimize the risk of a flare-up.

In addition, consider scheduling regular check-ins with yourself to assess your lifestyle choices. Are you managing stress effectively? Are you getting enough physical activity? Regularly evaluating these aspects can help you stay on track and reduce the chances of an unexpected gout attack.

Understanding Dietary and Lifestyle Factors Is Crucial

Diet plays a pivotal role in managing gout symptoms. Foods high in purines can elevate uric acid levels, so aim to incorporate low-purine options into your meals.

Focus on a diet rich in fruits, vegetables, whole grains, and low-fat dairy products. Foods like cherries and coffee may also help lower uric acid levels, making them beneficial choices.

Lifestyle factors, such as maintaining a healthy weight and exercising regularly, are equally important. Incorporate activities you enjoy, whether it's walking, cycling, or swimming, to make exercise a sustainable part of your routine. Additionally, aim for at least 30 minutes of moderate exercise most days to help manage weight and improve overall health, which can alleviate gout symptoms.

Importance of Consulting with Healthcare Professionals

Consulting with healthcare professionals is vital for managing gout effectively. Your primary care physician can provide a diagnosis and develop a personalized treatment plan based on your unique situation. They may recommend medications to lower uric acid levels and prevent attacks, as well as regular monitoring to ensure the treatment is effective.

In addition, consider seeking advice from a registered dietitian. They can help you create a customized meal plan that aligns with your dietary needs while keeping gout triggers in mind. Working collaboratively with healthcare professionals empowers you to make informed decisions and enhances your overall management of gout.

Overview of the Relationship Between Gout and Overall Health

Understanding the relationship between gout and your overall health is crucial for effective management. Gout is often associated with conditions such as obesity, hypertension, and cardiovascular disease. Recognizing this connection encourages a holistic approach to your health by addressing underlying conditions that may exacerbate gout.

Incorporate lifestyle changes that promote overall wellness, such as maintaining a balanced diet, engaging in regular physical activity, and managing stress. By improving your general health, you may also lower the frequency and severity of gout attacks. Regular check-ups with your healthcare provider can help you monitor your health status and make necessary adjustments to your management plan.

CHAPTER 1:

Causes of Gout

Explanation of Hyperuricemia (High Uric Acid Levels)

Hyperuricemia occurs when there are elevated levels of uric acid in the bloodstream, often due to overproduction or under-excretion by the kidneys. This condition is a precursor to gout, as excess uric acid can crystallize in joints, leading to painful inflammation. Monitoring uric acid levels through blood tests is essential for understanding an individual's risk of developing gout.

To manage hyperuricemia, individuals should aim to lower uric acid levels through dietary changes, medication, and lifestyle modifications. Regular check-ups with a healthcare provider can help track uric acid levels and implement necessary strategies, such as adjusting medication dosages or introducing uric acid-lowering drugs like allopurinol, which inhibits uric acid production.

Role of Genetics in Gout Predisposition

Genetics play a significant role in determining an individual's risk for gout. Studies have identified several genetic variants associated with how the body processes uric acid, making some people more susceptible to hyperuricemia and, consequently, gout attacks. Understanding family history can help assess risk levels.

To mitigate genetic predisposition, individuals can adopt a proactive approach by maintaining a healthy lifestyle and engaging in preventive measures. Genetic counseling may also be beneficial for those with a family history of gout, as it can provide insights into potential risks and management strategies tailored to an individual's genetic background.

Impact of Diet: Purine-Rich Foods to Avoid

Certain foods high in purines can elevate uric acid levels and trigger gout attacks. Common culprits include red meat, organ meats, shellfish, and certain fish, such as sardines and mackerel. It is crucial for individuals at risk of gout to be aware of these foods and limit their intake to help prevent flare-ups.

A practical approach to dietary management involves replacing purine-rich foods with alternatives that are lower in purines, such as fruits, vegetables, whole grains, and low-fat dairy products. Staying hydrated and incorporating complex carbohydrates can also help manage uric acid levels and support overall health.

Effects of Dehydration on Uric Acid Concentration

Dehydration can lead to increased uric acid concentration in the blood, as less water means less uric acid is excreted by the kidneys. Staying adequately hydrated is vital for those at risk of gout, as dehydration can trigger flare-ups and exacerbate symptoms. Drinking sufficient water daily is essential to maintain proper hydration levels.

To combat dehydration, individuals should aim to drink at least eight 8-ounce glasses of water daily, adjusting based on activity levels and climate. Incorporating hydrating foods, such as fruits and vegetables, can also support hydration and help dilute uric acid in the bloodstream.

Medical Conditions that Can Trigger Gout

Certain medical conditions, such as hypertension, diabetes, and kidney disease, can increase the risk of gout by affecting uric acid metabolism and excretion. Managing these underlying health issues is crucial for preventing gout attacks and maintaining overall health. Regular medical check-ups can help monitor these conditions.

Individuals should work closely with healthcare providers to address any existing medical conditions that may contribute to gout risk. Treatment plans may include lifestyle changes, medication adjustments, and ongoing monitoring of both uric acid levels and associated health issues to prevent complications.

Influence of Certain Medications on Uric Acid Levels

Some medications can raise uric acid levels, increasing the risk of gout. Common examples include diuretics (water pills), aspirin, and certain immunosuppressant's. It is essential for individuals to be aware of their medications and discuss any concerns with their healthcare provider.

To manage this risk, patients should review their medication regimen with their doctors. If necessary, healthcare providers may suggest alternative medications or adjustments that can help lower uric acid levels while still effectively treating other health conditions.

Lifestyle Factors such as Alcohol Consumption

Alcohol consumption, particularly beer and spirits, can increase uric acid production and decrease its elimination, contributing to gout flare-ups. It is advisable for individuals at risk of gout to limit or avoid alcohol intake to help manage their condition effectively.

To implement this change, individuals can start by tracking their alcohol consumption and gradually reducing intake. Opting for non-alcoholic beverages or low-purine drinks, like light wines, can also support uric acid management while maintaining social interactions.

The Role of Obesity in Increasing Gout Risk

Obesity is a significant risk factor for gout, as excess body weight can lead to increased uric acid production and decreased excretion. Managing body weight through a balanced diet and regular exercise is essential for those at risk of gout.

Individuals can adopt practical strategies to achieve a healthy weight, such as setting realistic weight loss goals, incorporating physical activity into daily routines, and making dietary changes that focus on nutrient-dense foods. Collaborating with a healthcare provider or nutritionist can provide additional support and guidance for sustainable weight management.

Hormonal Factors Affecting Uric Acid Production

Hormones, particularly estrogen, influence uric acid levels in the body. Women typically have lower uric acid levels before menopause due to estrogen's protective effects, but levels may rise after menopause. Understanding these hormonal changes can help individuals anticipate gout risk at different life stages.

To manage hormone-related changes, individuals should engage in regular physical activity, maintain a healthy diet, and monitor their uric acid levels, especially as they age. Consulting with a healthcare provider can provide insights into hormonal health and its impact on gout risk.

Impact of Age and Sex on Gout Occurrence

Gout is more common in men than women, largely due to hormonal differences, but the risk increases for both sexes with age. As individuals age, kidney function may decline, affecting uric acid elimination. Understanding this demographic factor can help individuals recognize their susceptibility to gout.

To address age-related risk, older adults should be vigilant about lifestyle factors that influence uric acid levels, such as diet and hydration. Regular health screenings can help catch elevated uric acid levels early, allowing for prompt management to prevent gout attacks.

Stress as a Potential Trigger for Gout Flare-Ups

Stress can exacerbate gout symptoms by increasing inflammation and potentially affecting uric acid levels. Finding effective ways to manage stress is crucial for individuals with a history of gout. Techniques such as mindfulness, yoga, and relaxation exercises can help reduce stress levels.

Incorporating stress management practices into daily routines can make a significant difference in preventing gout flare-ups. Setting aside time for relaxation and self-care, as well as seeking support from friends or professionals, can enhance emotional well-being and overall health.

Effects of High-Fructose Corn Syrup on Uric Acid Levels

High-fructose corn syrup (HFCS), commonly found in sugary beverages and processed foods, can lead to increased uric acid production. Limiting intake of HFCS can help manage uric acid levels and reduce the risk of gout attacks. Reading food labels and being aware of dietary sources of HFCS is crucial.

Individuals should focus on a diet rich in whole foods while avoiding sugary drinks and processed snacks high in HFCS. Choosing natural sweeteners, like honey or maple syrup, in moderation can also help maintain better control over uric acid levels.

Importance of Monitoring Kidney Function

Kidney function plays a critical role in uric acid excretion. Impaired kidney function can lead to increased uric acid levels and a higher risk of gout. Regular kidney function tests can help identify any potential issues and guide necessary lifestyle or medication changes.

To ensure optimal kidney health, individuals should stay well-hydrated, maintain a balanced diet low in processed foods, and manage underlying conditions such as diabetes or hypertension. Consulting with a healthcare provider about routine kidney function monitoring is essential for preventing complications associated with gout.

CHAPTER 2:

Symptoms of Gout

Sudden Onset of Intense Joint Pain

Gout often presents as a sudden and severe pain in the affected joint, typically starting during the night or early morning. This pain can be so intense that even the weight of a bed sheet may feel unbearable. It's crucial for individuals to recognize this intense pain as a potential symptom of gout, prompting them to seek medical attention promptly.

To manage this sudden pain effectively, the application of ice packs can provide immediate relief. Additionally, elevating the affected joint and resting it can help reduce pain levels. Over-the-counter nonsteroidal anti-inflammatory drugs (NSAIDs) like ibuprofen may also assist in alleviating discomfort, but it's advisable to consult a healthcare professional for a personalized treatment plan.

Redness and Swelling Around the Affected Joint

Redness and swelling are hallmark signs of a gout attack, often accompanied by an inflammatory response in the joint. The skin around the affected area may appear shiny and feel warm to the touch, indicating inflammation. This symptom signifies that the body is responding to elevated uric acid levels, which can lead to joint damage if not addressed.

To manage redness and swelling, consider taking anti-inflammatory medications as directed by a healthcare provider. Maintaining a cool compress on the joint can also help reduce inflammation. Staying hydrated is essential, as adequate fluid intake helps flush uric acid from the body, potentially preventing future attacks.

Warmth in the Affected Area

During a gout flare-up, the affected joint often feels warm, a sign of inflammation. This warmth results from increased blood flow to the area as the body fights off the buildup of uric acid crystals. Recognizing this symptom early can help individuals understand they are experiencing a gout attack, guiding them toward appropriate treatment.

To alleviate warmth and discomfort, applying a cold compress to the joint can help reduce swelling and provide soothing relief. It's also beneficial to avoid strenuous activities that may exacerbate inflammation during an active flare-up, allowing the joint to rest and heal.

Morning Stiffness After an Attack

Many individuals with gout experience stiffness in the affected joint upon waking after an attack. This stiffness can hinder mobility and make everyday activities challenging. It often signifies lingering inflammation, which can be distressing for those already coping with acute pain.

To manage morning stiffness, gentle stretching exercises or range-of-motion activities can help restore flexibility. Additionally, soaking the affected joint in warm water or applying heat may ease stiffness, making it easier to move throughout the day. Regularly incorporating low-impact exercises can also prevent stiffness in the long term.

Duration and Pattern of Pain during Flare-Ups

Gout flare-ups can vary in duration, typically lasting from a few days to a couple of weeks. Understanding the pattern of pain can be helpful for individuals to anticipate and manage their symptoms effectively. Pain often begins suddenly, peaks within 24 hours, and gradually subsides, but recurrent episodes can occur if the underlying causes are not addressed.

Keeping a pain diary can assist individuals in tracking the duration and intensity of their symptoms. This information can be valuable when consulting with a healthcare provider, as it helps determine the most effective treatment and management strategies for future attacks.

Commonly Affected Joints (e.g., Big Toe)

Gout most frequently affects the big toe, but other joints such as the ankles, knees, and fingers can also be involved. Recognizing which joints are commonly affected can aid in early identification and management of gout. The first metatarsophalangeal joint, located at the base of the big toe, is particularly susceptible to gout attacks.

To manage symptoms in affected joints, individuals can benefit from rest and immobilization during flare-ups. Applying ice or a cold pack can help reduce pain and swelling, while maintaining an appropriate diet low in purines may minimize future occurrences.

Possible Fever Accompanying Severe Attacks

During severe gout attacks, some individuals may experience a mild fever. This fever is a sign of inflammation and indicates that the body is responding to the presence of uric acid crystals. Monitoring body temperature during an attack can help individuals assess the severity of their condition.

If fever occurs, it's essential to consult a healthcare provider for evaluation and treatment options. Staying hydrated and resting can support recovery, while over-the-counter medications may be recommended to alleviate both pain and fever.

Difficulty Moving the Affected Joint

A common symptom of gout is difficulty moving the affected joint due to pain and swelling. This limitation can impact daily activities, making it challenging to perform tasks that require joint mobility. Recognizing this symptom is crucial for understanding the extent of the gout attack.

To manage joint mobility, gentle range-of-motion exercises can help maintain flexibility. Engaging in physical therapy may also provide guidance on specific exercises tailored to individual needs, promoting better movement and reducing stiffness.

Chronic Symptoms vs. Acute Flare-Ups

Gout can present both chronic symptoms and acute flare-ups. Chronic gout may involve persistent discomfort and sensitivity in the affected joints, while acute flare-ups are characterized by sudden, intense pain. Understanding the distinction between these symptoms can assist individuals in managing their condition effectively.

For chronic symptoms, lifestyle changes such as maintaining a healthy weight and adhering to a low-purine diet can significantly improve quality of life. On the other hand, acute flare-ups require prompt attention and may benefit from medications prescribed by a healthcare professional to reduce pain and inflammation.

Potential for Developing Tophi (Deposits of Uric Acid)

Individuals with untreated gout may develop tophi, which are deposits of uric acid crystals that can form under the skin, usually around joints. These lumps can be painful and may indicate chronic gout, signaling the need for more effective management strategies. Recognizing the potential for tophi can motivate individuals to take preventive measures.

To minimize the risk of developing tophi, it's crucial to maintain a well-managed diet and stay hydrated. Regular medical check-ups can help monitor uric acid levels, and healthcare providers may prescribe medications to keep these levels within a healthy range, preventing the formation of tophi.

Recurrent Attacks and Their Frequency

Gout is characterized by recurrent attacks that can vary in frequency from several times a year to infrequent episodes. Understanding the frequency of attacks is essential for individuals to develop effective management plans. Regular flare-ups may indicate uncontrolled uric acid levels, necessitating lifestyle and dietary adjustments.

To reduce the frequency of attacks, individuals should focus on long-term lifestyle changes, such as maintaining a balanced diet, exercising regularly, and managing stress. Consulting a healthcare professional for a tailored plan can also help identify triggers and establish preventative strategies.

Importance of Recognizing Symptoms Early

Early recognition of gout symptoms is vital for effective management and prevention of severe flare-ups. Individuals who can identify the initial signs, such as sudden joint pain and swelling, are better positioned to take prompt action, which can mitigate the severity of an attack.

Keeping a symptom diary and being aware of personal triggers can aid in early detection. By understanding their unique patterns of symptoms, individuals can work with healthcare providers to create proactive management strategies, ultimately reducing the impact of gout on their daily lives.

Differentiating Gout from Other Types of Arthritis

Gout can sometimes be mistaken for other types of arthritis, making accurate diagnosis crucial. Key differences include the sudden onset and intensity of pain in gout compared to the more gradual symptoms of other forms of arthritis. Recognizing these distinctions can guide individuals toward appropriate treatment options.

For an accurate diagnosis, individuals should consult healthcare providers who may perform blood tests, joint fluid analysis, or imaging studies.

CHAPTER 3:

Diagnosis of Gout

Importance of Medical History in Diagnosis

A comprehensive medical history is crucial in diagnosing gout as it provides insights into the patient's previous health conditions, lifestyle, and family history of gout or related disorders. Patients should discuss their symptoms, including the onset, duration, and frequency of joint pain, swelling, and any associated factors such as recent dietary changes or medications. This information helps healthcare providers identify patterns that could indicate gout.

During the medical history evaluation, the doctor may inquire about the patient's diet, alcohol consumption, and any medications that could affect uric acid levels, such as diuretics. By understanding these factors, healthcare professionals can better assess the likelihood of gout and decide on further diagnostic steps.

Physical Examination by a Healthcare Professional

A thorough physical examination is essential in diagnosing gout, focusing on the affected joints. The healthcare provider will inspect and palpate the joints for signs of swelling, redness, and tenderness, particularly in common gout-affected areas like the big toe, knees, and ankles. The degree of pain experienced during the examination can help indicate the severity of the condition.

Additionally, the clinician may assess the range of motion in the affected joints and look for other physical signs that could suggest gout or related conditions. This hands-on evaluation complements the medical history and guides the decision-making process for further diagnostic testing.

Joint Aspiration to Analyze Synovial Fluid

Joint aspiration, or arthrocentesis, involves using a sterile needle to withdraw synovial fluid from the affected joint. This procedure is performed by a healthcare professional and can provide immediate relief from pain and swelling while allowing for laboratory analysis of the fluid. The presence of uric acid crystals in the fluid is a definitive sign of gout.

To prepare for the procedure, the patient should remain still and may be given local anesthesia to minimize discomfort. After fluid extraction, the sample is sent to a laboratory where it is examined under a microscope, helping to confirm a gout diagnosis or rule out other conditions.

Blood Tests to Measure Uric Acid Levels

Blood tests are critical for measuring serum uric acid levels, as elevated levels are commonly associated with gout. A healthcare provider will draw blood from the patient, typically from a vein in the arm, and send the sample for analysis. Understanding these levels aids in diagnosing gout and assessing the severity of the condition.

It's essential for patients to fast for at least four hours before the blood test for accurate results. If uric acid levels are high, the healthcare provider may recommend further tests or lifestyle changes to help manage uric acid levels and prevent future gout attacks.

Imaging Studies (e.g., X-rays) to Assess Joint Damage

Imaging studies like X-rays are used to evaluate joint damage caused by gout. While X-rays cannot directly visualize uric acid crystals, they help identify changes in joint structure, such as erosion or joint space narrowing, which may occur over time with untreated gout. These findings can provide valuable information about the progression of the disease.

Patients should inform their healthcare provider about any allergies to contrast materials if a more detailed imaging study, like a CT scan or MRI, is needed. By monitoring changes through imaging, healthcare providers can adjust treatment strategies effectively to minimize long-term joint damage.

Differential Diagnosis to Rule Out Other Conditions

Differential diagnosis is a process where healthcare professionals rule out other potential conditions that may mimic gout symptoms, such as rheumatoid arthritis, pseudo gout, or septic arthritis. This step is essential to ensure that the treatment provided addresses the correct diagnosis. Physicians will consider the patient's medical history, physical examination results, and any laboratory findings during this process.

To carry out a differential diagnosis, healthcare providers may order additional tests or imaging studies to evaluate other potential causes of joint pain and inflammation. By systematically ruling out these alternatives, providers can confidently diagnose gout and implement an effective treatment plan.

Understanding the Role of a Healthcare Team

A healthcare team typically consists of various professionals, including primary care physicians, rheumatologists, dietitians, and physical therapists, all contributing to the management of gout. Each team member plays a vital role in assessing, diagnosing, and treating the condition, ensuring a comprehensive approach to patient care.

For effective management, patients should communicate openly with each team member about their symptoms, treatment responses, and lifestyle changes. Collaboration among healthcare professionals enhances the quality of care, allowing for tailored treatment strategies that address the individual needs of the patient.

Importance of Accurate Diagnosis for Effective Treatment

An accurate diagnosis is critical in managing gout effectively, as it guides treatment decisions and helps prevent future flare-ups. Misdiagnosis can lead to inappropriate treatments that may exacerbate symptoms or cause unwanted side effects. Thus, thorough diagnostic procedures and discussions between the patient and healthcare provider are essential.

Once gout is accurately diagnosed, treatment plans can include medications to lower uric acid levels, lifestyle modifications, and dietary changes. By establishing a correct diagnosis, healthcare professionals can optimize patient outcomes and improve quality of life.

Monitoring Changes in Symptoms over Time

Monitoring changes in symptoms is vital for individuals with gout, as it allows for timely adjustments to treatment strategies. Patients should keep a symptom diary, noting the frequency, intensity, and duration of gout attacks, as well as any triggers such as diet or stress. This record can help healthcare providers assess the effectiveness of treatment and make necessary adjustments.

Regular follow-ups with a healthcare provider are essential to review the symptom diary and discuss any changes in condition. Through ongoing monitoring, patients can better manage their gout and reduce the risk of severe flare-ups.

Use of Ultrasound to Detect Uric Acid Crystals

Ultrasound is a non-invasive imaging technique used to visualize uric acid crystals in joints and soft tissues. This method is particularly beneficial in diagnosing gout, as it can identify early changes and deposits of crystals that may not yet have caused visible damage. During the procedure, a gel is applied to the skin, and a transducer is moved over the area to capture images.

Patients should follow any pre-procedure instructions provided by their healthcare provider, such as avoiding food or drink beforehand. The results from the ultrasound can aid in confirming a gout diagnosis and help shape a comprehensive management plan.

Biopsy in Rare Cases to Confirm Gout

A biopsy is a procedure in which a small sample of tissue is taken from the affected area to determine the presence of uric acid crystals or other abnormalities. While not common for diagnosing gout, it may be performed in rare or complex cases where the diagnosis is unclear. The procedure typically requires local anesthesia, and the tissue sample is sent to a laboratory for analysis.

Patients should discuss the risks and benefits of a biopsy with their healthcare provider, who will explain the procedure and provide aftercare instructions. In cases where gout is confirmed, the biopsy results can help guide effective treatment strategies.

Role of Patient Education in Diagnosis

Patient education plays a crucial role in the diagnosis and management of gout. Patients should be informed about the disease, its symptoms, and potential triggers to facilitate early detection. Understanding how lifestyle choices, such as diet and hydration, affect uric acid levels empowers individuals to make informed decisions that can prevent gout attacks.

Healthcare providers should offer resources, such as pamphlets or workshops, to educate patients about gout management. By actively participating in their care, patients can improve their understanding of the condition and enhance their ability to communicate effectively with their healthcare team.

Regular Check-ups for Chronic Sufferers

Regular check-ups are essential for individuals with chronic gout to monitor their condition and adjust treatment plans as necessary. During these appointments, healthcare providers will review the patient's medical history, assess symptoms, and conduct relevant tests to evaluate uric acid levels and joint health. These proactive measures can help prevent flare-ups and complications.

Patients should schedule routine appointments, even when symptoms are well-managed, to ensure ongoing care. By maintaining open communication with their healthcare team, individuals can effectively manage their gout and improve their overall quality of life.

CHAPTER 4:

Effective Management Strategies

Role of Medication in Managing Gout (e.g., NSAIDs)

Medications, particularly nonsteroidal anti-inflammatory drugs (NSAIDs), play a crucial role in managing gout by alleviating pain and reducing inflammation during acute attacks. Common NSAIDs include ibuprofen and naproxen, which can help manage flare-ups effectively. For optimal results, it's essential to start taking NSAIDs as soon as symptoms begin, and they should be taken as directed by a healthcare professional to minimize side effects.

In addition to NSAIDs, other medications like colchicines can also be effective in treating gout attacks by decreasing inflammation. Understanding how these medications work and following your healthcare provider's guidance will ensure a smoother recovery and help prevent future attacks.

Importance of Following Prescribed Treatment Plans

Following prescribed treatment plans is vital for effectively managing gout and preventing future flare-ups. Adherence to medication schedules, including urate-lowering therapy, helps maintain lower uric acid levels, which is essential in preventing gout attacks. Patients should communicate openly with their healthcare providers about any difficulties they face in following their treatment plans to receive the necessary adjustments and support.

Moreover, being consistent with treatment not only alleviates symptoms but also contributes to long-term health. Patients should keep a medication diary to track doses and timings, making it easier to stay on course and recognize patterns in their treatment efficacy.

Use of Corticosteroids for Severe Attacks

Corticosteroids are often prescribed for severe gout attacks when NSAIDs are ineffective or contraindicated. These medications work by quickly reducing inflammation and pain, providing relief to patients who experience debilitating symptoms. Corticosteroids can be administered orally or through injections, depending on the severity of the attack and the patient's specific situation.

It's essential to use corticosteroids under a healthcare provider's supervision due to potential side effects with long-term use. Patients should discuss their symptoms and treatment options with their doctors to determine the best course of action for managing acute gout flares effectively.

Introduction of Urate-Lowering Therapy (ULT)

Urate-lowering therapy (ULT) is a long-term management strategy aimed at reducing uric acid levels in the blood, which is crucial for preventing future gout attacks. Medications such as allopurinol or febuxostat are commonly prescribed ULT options. Patients typically start on a low dose, gradually increasing it under medical supervision until target uric acid levels are achieved.

Adopting ULT is essential for those experiencing recurrent gout attacks. Regular follow-ups with healthcare providers will help ensure that uric acid levels are monitored and maintained within the desired range, significantly reducing the risk of future episodes.

Lifestyle Modifications for Effective Management

Making lifestyle modifications can significantly enhance the effectiveness of gout management. Patients should focus on maintaining a balanced diet, incorporating whole foods, and avoiding high-purine foods such as red meat, organ meats, and shellfish. Simple changes, like substituting processed foods with fresh fruits and vegetables, can contribute to overall health and help control gout.

Additionally, managing stress through relaxation techniques such as yoga or meditation can positively impact gout symptoms. Small, manageable changes, like preparing meals at home and scheduling regular physical activity, can foster a sustainable lifestyle that supports effective gout management.

Importance of Regular Monitoring of Uric Acid Levels

Regular monitoring of uric acid levels is vital in managing gout effectively. Patients should have routine blood tests to check their uric acid levels, ensuring they remain within the target range set by their healthcare provider. This proactive approach helps to assess the effectiveness of current treatments and make necessary adjustments.

Keeping track of uric acid levels also helps patients understand their condition better and identify factors that may trigger flare-ups. Utilizing a health app or a journal can simplify this process, allowing patients to log their results and discuss them during medical appointments.

Staying Hydrated to Help Flush Uric Acid

Staying hydrated is a fundamental yet often overlooked aspect of managing gout. Drinking plenty of water helps dilute uric acid in the bloodstream and promotes its elimination through urine. Aiming for at least eight to ten glasses of water a day can aid in flushing excess uric acid from the body.

In addition to water, patients can include hydrating foods like fruits and vegetables in their diet. Consuming herbal teas or broths can also contribute to hydration while providing additional nutrients that support overall health.

Dietary Adjustments: What to Include and Avoid

Making dietary adjustments is key to managing gout effectively. Patients should focus on including low-purine foods in their diet, such as whole grains, low-fat dairy, fruits, and vegetables. Incorporating foods rich in vitamin C, like oranges and strawberries, can also help lower uric acid levels.

Conversely, individuals should avoid foods high in purines, including red meat, organ meats, and certain seafood like sardines and mussels. Reducing alcohol consumption, especially beer, is equally important, as it can raise uric acid levels and increase the risk of flare-ups.

Regular Exercise as a Part of the Management Plan

Regular exercise plays a crucial role in managing gout by helping to maintain a healthy weight and reduce stress levels. Engaging in low-impact activities, such as walking, swimming, or cycling, can promote cardiovascular health without putting excess strain on joints. Aiming for at least 30 minutes of moderate exercise most days of the week can yield significant benefits.

Incorporating strength training exercises twice a week can further enhance muscle tone and support joint health. Developing a consistent exercise routine not only improves physical fitness but also helps manage weight, ultimately contributing to lower uric acid levels and fewer gout attacks.

Weight Loss Strategies for Overweight Individuals

For individuals with gout who are overweight, weight loss can significantly reduce the frequency and severity of attacks. Implementing gradual changes to diet and exercise is key; aiming for a loss of 1 to 2 pounds per week is generally considered safe and sustainable. Focusing on portion control and choosing nutrient-dense foods can aid in achieving weight loss goals.

Combining dietary changes with regular physical activity creates a comprehensive approach to weight loss. Working with a healthcare provider or nutritionist can provide tailored strategies, making it easier to stay motivated and on track with weight loss efforts.

Support Groups and Counseling for Emotional Support

Support groups and counseling can be invaluable resources for individuals managing gout. Connecting with others facing similar challenges can provide emotional support and practical advice. Many communities offer in-person or online support groups where individuals can share experiences and coping strategies.

Additionally, seeking counseling can help patients address the emotional aspects of living with a chronic condition like gout. A therapist can assist in developing coping mechanisms and strategies for managing stress, which can ultimately improve overall well-being and adherence to treatment plans.

Importance of Tracking Symptoms and Triggers

Tracking symptoms and triggers is essential for effective gout management. Keeping a detailed log of symptoms, dietary habits, physical activity, and flare-ups can help identify patterns and potential triggers. Patients can use a journal or mobile apps to document this information, making it easier to recognize what may contribute to their condition.

Understanding personal triggers, such as specific foods or activities, empowers patients to make informed decisions that can help prevent future attacks.

Building a Personal Gout Management Plan

Creating a personal gout management plan is crucial for maintaining control over the condition. This plan should include medication schedules, dietary guidelines, exercise routines, and hydration strategies tailored to the individual's needs. Collaborating with healthcare providers ensures the plan is comprehensive and effective.

Patients should regularly reassess and update their management plans based on changes in symptoms or lifestyle. Setting realistic goals and tracking progress can provide motivation and help maintain long-term adherence to the plan, ultimately leading to improved health outcomes.

CHAPTER 5:

Dietary Considerations

Overview of Foods High in Purines to Avoid

Foods high in purines can significantly elevate uric acid levels in the body, leading to gout attacks. Key foods to avoid include red meats, organ meats (like liver), and certain seafood (such as sardines and anchovies). These foods should be minimized or eliminated from your diet to help manage and prevent gout flare-ups.

In addition to meats and seafood, high-purine foods also include certain legumes and some vegetables, such as asparagus and spinach. Understanding which foods to avoid is crucial for anyone looking to manage their gout effectively. Reading labels and being mindful of meal choices can make a significant difference.

List of Low-Purine Food Options

Low-purine foods are essential for managing gout, providing a safe way to enjoy meals without triggering symptoms. Opt for low-fat dairy products, eggs, and a variety of fruits and vegetables. Foods like cherries, which may even help lower uric acid levels, are particularly beneficial.

In addition to fruits and vegetables, consider incorporating whole grains, such as brown rice, quinoa, and oats, into your diet. These foods not only provide essential nutrients but also help in maintaining a balanced diet that supports overall health while managing gout effectively.

Importance of a Balanced Diet for Overall Health

A balanced diet plays a crucial role in maintaining overall health and preventing chronic conditions, including gout. It is essential to include a variety of food groups, such as fruits, vegetables, whole grains, lean proteins, and healthy fats, to ensure that your body receives all necessary nutrients.

By following a balanced diet, you can support your immune system, maintain a healthy weight, and reduce inflammation, all of which are critical for managing gout. Meal planning and preparation can help you stick to your dietary goals and avoid triggers that could lead to flare-ups.

Role of Dairy Products in Reducing Gout Risk

Dairy products, especially low-fat options, can play a significant role in reducing the risk of gout. Studies suggest that consuming low-fat milk and yogurt can lower uric acid levels and potentially prevent gout attacks. Aim for at least one serving of low-fat dairy per day as part of your diet.

Incorporating dairy into your meals is simple; use yogurt as a base for smoothies or dress salads with a light yogurt dressing. Cheese can also be included in moderation. These small changes can help maintain healthy uric acid levels and provide essential nutrients.

Hydration Strategies and Their Impact on Uric Acid

Staying hydrated is vital for managing gout, as it helps to dilute uric acid levels in the blood and promotes its excretion through urine. Aim to drink at least eight glasses of water per day, and consider increasing your intake during hot weather or physical activity.

Herbal teas and infused water with fruits like lemon or cucumber can also be excellent hydration options. Avoiding dehydrating beverages, such as caffeinated drinks and alcohol, will further help manage uric acid levels effectively.

Benefits of Whole Grains and Vegetables

Whole grains and vegetables are key components of a diet that helps manage gout. Whole grains like brown rice, quinoa, and whole wheat bread provide fiber, which supports digestive health and can aid in weight management. Including a variety of colorful vegetables ensures you get essential vitamins and antioxidants.

Incorporate at least three servings of vegetables into your daily meals, experimenting with different cooking methods such as steaming or roasting to enhance their flavor. These foods not only provide nutrients but also help reduce the overall purine content of your diet.

Understanding the Impact of Sugar-Sweetened Beverages

Sugar-sweetened beverages, particularly those high in fructose, can lead to increased uric acid levels and trigger gout attacks. It is essential to limit or eliminate sodas and other sweetened drinks from your diet. Opt for water, herbal teas, or naturally flavored seltzer as healthier alternatives.

Reading nutritional labels on beverages can help you avoid hidden sugars. By making these small changes, you can significantly lower your risk of gout flare-ups and improve your overall health.

Alcohol: Which Types to Avoid and Which May Be Safer

Alcohol consumption can impact uric acid levels, making some drinks more problematic than others. Beer and distilled liquors are typically high in purines and should be avoided. If you choose to drink, opt for light to moderate consumption of wine, which may be a safer choice for those managing gout.

Monitor your alcohol intake closely and try to limit your consumption to special occasions. Keeping track of your reactions to different types of alcohol can help you identify what works for your body and what doesn't.

Importance of Portion Control in Meals

Portion control is crucial for managing gout, as overeating can lead to weight gain, which increases uric acid levels. Practicing portion control involves measuring servings and being mindful of portion sizes at meals. Use smaller plates or bowls to help manage portions more effectively.

Taking the time to enjoy your meals can also help prevent overeating. Eating slowly and paying attention to hunger cues allows your body to signal when it's full, helping you maintain a healthy weight and manage gout symptoms more effectively.

Nutritional Supplements That May Help Manage Gout

Certain nutritional supplements may aid in managing gout symptoms and lowering uric acid levels. Vitamin C has been shown to help reduce uric acid, while fish oil supplements can provide anti-inflammatory benefits. Always consult with a healthcare provider before starting any new supplement regimen.

In addition to supplements, incorporating foods rich in these nutrients can also be beneficial. Foods like citrus fruits, fatty fish, and walnuts can help support your overall health while potentially reducing the risk of gout flare-ups.

Planning Meals to Avoid Gout Triggers

Meal planning is an effective strategy for avoiding gout triggers and ensuring a balanced diet. Create a weekly meal plan that includes low-purine foods, focusing on whole grains, fruits, and vegetables. Prepare meals in advance to avoid last-minute unhealthy choices.

Incorporating a variety of flavors and cooking methods can keep your meals exciting while adhering to dietary guidelines. Use herbs and spices to enhance the taste of your dishes, making it easier to stick to your meal plan.

Keeping a Food Diary to Track Symptoms

Maintaining a food diary can help you identify specific foods that trigger gout symptoms. Record everything you eat and drink, along with any symptoms you experience. Over time, this can reveal patterns that help you avoid specific triggers.

Reviewing your food diary regularly can help you make informed dietary choices. It can also be a useful tool when discussing your condition with healthcare providers or dietitians, enabling them to offer personalized recommendations based on your findings.

Consulting with a Registered Dietitian for Personalized Advice

Consulting with a registered dietitian can provide invaluable support in managing gout. A dietitian can help you create a tailored meal plan that considers your dietary preferences, health goals, and any specific triggers you may have. This personalized approach can make a significant difference in managing your condition.

Working with a dietitian also allows for ongoing support and adjustments to your plan as needed. They can provide education on nutrition and help you develop sustainable eating habits that promote overall health while managing gout effectively.

CHAPTER 6:

Lifestyle Changes for Prevention

Importance of Maintaining a Healthy Weight

Maintaining a healthy weight is crucial for preventing gout attacks, as excess weight increases uric acid levels in the blood. Achieving a healthy weight can be done by calculating your body mass index (BMI) and setting realistic weight loss goals. Aim for gradual weight loss through balanced nutrition and regular exercise, focusing on nutrient-dense foods while reducing caloric intake.

To maintain your weight, consider meal prepping to control portion sizes and make healthier choices. Incorporate more fruits, vegetables, whole grains, and lean proteins into your diet while reducing processed foods high in sugars and fats. Regularly monitor your weight and adjust your diet and exercise routine as necessary to stay within your target range.

Regular Physical Activity and Its Benefits

Engaging in regular physical activity can significantly reduce the risk of gout attacks by helping to lower uric acid levels. Aim for at least 150 minutes of moderate-intensity aerobic exercise weekly, such as brisk walking, cycling, or swimming. Incorporate strength training exercises at least two days a week to enhance muscle mass and metabolism.

In addition to preventing gout, physical activity improves overall health by promoting heart health, improving joint mobility, and reducing stress. Start with small, manageable goals, like a daily 10-minute walk, and gradually increase intensity and duration as you build stamina. Finding an enjoyable activity can also help you stay motivated and consistent.

Stress Management Techniques (e.g., Meditation)

Stress can trigger gout attacks, so practicing stress management techniques is vital. One effective method is meditation, which involves focusing your mind and calming your thoughts. To get started, find a quiet space, sit comfortably, and close your eyes. Focus on your breath, inhaling deeply and exhaling slowly, allowing distractions to fade away.

Incorporate short meditation sessions into your daily routine, gradually increasing the duration as you become more comfortable. Other stress management techniques include deep breathing exercises, yoga, and spending time in nature. Consistent practice can lead to improved emotional well-being and reduced stress levels, which may help in preventing gout flare-ups.

Importance of Hydration and Recommended Daily Intake

Staying hydrated is essential for preventing gout, as it helps to flush uric acid from the body. Aim for at least 8-10 cups of water daily, adjusting based on your activity level and climate. Keep a water bottle handy throughout the day to encourage regular hydration, and consider infusing water with fruits or herbs for added flavor.

Pay attention to signs of dehydration, such as dark urine or dry skin, and increase your fluid intake accordingly. Additionally, limit beverages that can contribute to dehydration, such as alcohol and sugary drinks, opting instead for water, herbal teas, or low-sugar options. Staying adequately hydrated can reduce the frequency of gout attacks.

Smoking Cessation as a Preventive Measure

Quitting smoking is an important step in reducing the risk of gout, as smoking can elevate uric acid levels and decrease the body's ability to eliminate it. To quit, set a quit date and create a plan that includes identifying triggers and finding healthy coping strategies. Seek support from friends, family, or professional resources to help you stay accountable.

Consider using nicotine replacement therapies, like patches or gums, to manage withdrawal symptoms. Engage in activities that keep your hands and mind occupied, such as exercising or picking up a new hobby. Celebrate your milestones along the way to maintain motivation and reduce the likelihood of relapse.

Incorporating Mindfulness in Daily Routines

Incorporating mindfulness into your daily routine can help reduce stress and promote emotional well-being, which may help manage gout symptoms. Start by practicing mindfulness during everyday activities, such as eating or walking. Focus on the sensory experiences, like the taste and texture of food or the sounds of nature, to cultivate present-moment awareness.

Set aside specific times each day for dedicated mindfulness practices, such as meditation or deep breathing exercises. Use apps or online resources to guide your practice if you're new to mindfulness. Consistency is key; even a few minutes daily can help you develop greater awareness and resilience, contributing to better overall health.

Establishing a Regular Sleep Schedule

A regular sleep schedule plays a crucial role in overall health and can help prevent gout flare-ups. Aim for 7-9 hours of quality sleep each night by going to bed and waking up at the same time daily. Create a relaxing bedtime routine that includes activities like reading, taking a warm bath, or practicing deep breathing to signal to your body that it's time to wind down.

Ensure your sleep environment is conducive to restful sleep by keeping your bedroom dark, quiet, and cool. Limit exposure to screens and blue light at least an hour before bedtime, and consider using blackout curtains or white noise machines to enhance your sleep quality. Prioritizing sleep can support your body's recovery and reduce inflammation, contributing to better management of gout.

Limiting Exposure to High-Fructose Corn Syrup

High-fructose corn syrup (HFCS) can increase uric acid levels and trigger gout attacks. To limit exposure, read food labels and avoid products with HFCS as an ingredient, commonly found in sugary beverages, processed snacks, and sweets. Instead, choose natural sweeteners like honey or pure maple syrup in moderation.

Focus on whole, unprocessed foods in your diet, such as fruits, vegetables, whole grains, and lean proteins. When craving something sweet, opt for fresh fruit instead of sugary snacks. Being mindful of your sugar intake can significantly impact your uric acid levels and overall health.

Understanding the Impact of Processed Foods

Processed foods often contain unhealthy fats, sugars, and additives that can contribute to increased uric acid levels and inflammation. To minimize their impact, prioritize whole foods over packaged items, preparing meals at home whenever possible. When shopping, opt for fresh ingredients and read labels carefully to choose items with minimal processing.

If you do consume processed foods, try to limit them to occasional treats rather than staples in your diet. Aim to incorporate more fruits, vegetables, whole grains, and lean proteins into your meals. By focusing on nourishing foods, you can support your body's health and potentially reduce the risk of gout attacks.

Social Support Networks for Lifestyle Changes

Having a strong social support network can significantly influence your success in making lifestyle changes to manage gout. Surround yourself with friends and family who encourage healthy habits, and consider joining support groups or online communities focused on gout management. Sharing experiences and challenges with others can provide motivation and accountability.

Engage in activities with supportive individuals, such as cooking healthy meals together or exercising as a group. Celebrate each other's successes and offer encouragement during difficult times. Building a network of support can make the journey to better health more enjoyable and sustainable.

Setting Achievable Health Goals

Setting achievable health goals is essential for successfully managing gout and promoting overall wellness. Start by identifying specific, measurable, and time-bound goals, such as losing a certain amount of weight, exercising for a specific duration, or increasing your water intake. Break larger goals into smaller, manageable steps to prevent feeling overwhelmed.

Regularly review your goals to track your progress and make adjustments as needed. Celebrate your achievements, no matter how small, to stay motivated. Having clear goals helps provide direction and focus, making it easier to implement lifestyle changes that support gout management.

Keeping Track of Progress Through Journaling

Keeping a journal can be a powerful tool for tracking your progress in managing gout. Record daily activities, dietary choices, stress levels, and symptoms to identify patterns and triggers. This reflection can help you make informed decisions about your lifestyle and adjust your habits accordingly.

Set aside time each day or week to review your journal entries and evaluate your progress toward your health goals. Use this information to celebrate successes, learn from challenges, and make necessary adjustments. Journaling can promote self-awareness and empower you to take control of your health journey.

Seeking Professional Help When Needed

When managing gout, seeking professional help can provide valuable guidance and support. If you experience frequent flare-ups or struggle with lifestyle changes, consider consulting a healthcare provider or a registered dietitian. They can help you develop a personalized plan that addresses your unique needs and concerns.

Don't hesitate to reach out for assistance when feeling overwhelmed or uncertain about your management strategies. Professional support can help you navigate the complexities of gout and provide evidence-based recommendations. Prioritizing your health is essential, and seeking help is a positive step toward better management.

CHAPTER 7:

Alternative Therapies

Overview of Herbal Remedies for Gout Relief

Herbal remedies can be effective in managing gout symptoms due to their natural anti-inflammatory and uric acid-lowering properties. Common herbs like ginger, turmeric, and devil's claw may help reduce swelling and pain. Incorporating these herbs into your diet, whether in tea, capsules, or food, can offer a complementary approach to traditional treatments.

To use herbal remedies effectively, start by researching each herb's proper dosage and potential side effects. Consider consulting with a qualified herbalist or healthcare provider to create a personalized plan that suits your needs. Keep a journal to track your symptoms and any changes you notice while using these remedies, ensuring you can adjust as necessary.

Benefits of Acupuncture in Pain Management

Acupuncture involves inserting thin needles into specific points on the body, which may help alleviate pain associated with gout. This technique is believed to enhance blood flow and release endorphins, providing a natural pain-relieving effect. Many individuals report reduced pain levels and increased mobility after a few sessions.

To incorporate acupuncture into your pain management plan, seek a licensed acupuncturist experienced in treating gout. Attend a consultation to discuss your symptoms and treatment goals, allowing the practitioner to tailor their approach. Regular sessions may lead to long-term relief, so commit to a schedule that aligns with your comfort and budget.

Exploring the Use of Homeopathy for Symptoms

Homeopathy offers individualized treatments that may help relieve gout symptoms by stimulating the body's natural healing processes. Remedies such as Colchicum and Rhododendron can target specific symptoms like pain and inflammation. These remedies are typically diluted and taken in pellet form, making them easy to administer.

To use homeopathy effectively, consult a professional homeopath who can assess your symptoms and recommend suitable remedies. Keep track of how you respond to the treatment, adjusting the dosage or remedy as needed. It's essential to remain patient, as homeopathic treatments may take time to show results.

Importance of Discussing Alternative Therapies with Doctors

Before starting any alternative therapies for gout relief, it's crucial to discuss your plans with your healthcare provider. This dialogue ensures that the alternative methods won't interfere with your existing treatments or exacerbate your condition. Open communication about your health goals can help your doctor guide you effectively.

Additionally, maintaining a collaborative relationship with your healthcare provider allows you to explore a holistic treatment plan that incorporates both traditional and alternative therapies. Keep your doctor informed about any changes you experience while trying these therapies, as they may adjust your medication or recommend further interventions.

Role of Physical Therapy in Recovery

Physical therapy plays a vital role in recovering from gout flare-ups by improving joint mobility and strengthening the surrounding muscles. A physical therapist can design a personalized exercise program that focuses on gentle stretching and strengthening, tailored to your specific needs and limitations.

Engage in regular sessions and perform prescribed exercises at home to enhance your recovery. Your therapist will monitor your progress and adjust the program as needed, helping you regain strength and flexibility while minimizing the risk of future flare-ups.

Benefits of Hot/Cold Therapy for Pain Relief

Hot and cold therapy can effectively manage gout pain and inflammation. Cold packs can numb the area and reduce swelling during flare-ups, while heat can relax muscles and improve blood circulation afterward. Apply a cold pack for 15-20 minutes during a flare and use heat, such as a warm towel or heating pad, for the same duration post-flare.

To implement this therapy, always protect your skin with a cloth to prevent burns or frostbite. Experiment with both methods to see which one offers more relief for your symptoms, and adjust your approach based on your body's response.

Investigating Supplements (e.g., Cherry Extract)

Supplements like cherry extract have gained attention for their potential to lower uric acid levels and reduce gout attacks. Research suggests that consuming cherry extract or whole cherries can help decrease inflammation and may be beneficial for gout sufferers. Taking these supplements regularly can provide additional support alongside traditional treatments.

To incorporate cherry extract into your routine, look for high-quality products that specify the concentration of anthocyanins, the active compounds thought to provide relief. Follow the recommended dosage on the product label, and consult with your healthcare provider to ensure it aligns with your overall treatment plan.

Use of Essential Oils for Topical Relief

Essential oils such as lavender, peppermint, and eucalyptus possess anti-inflammatory properties that may help alleviate gout pain when applied topically. Diluting essential oils with a carrier oil (like coconut or olive oil) and massaging the mixture onto affected joints can provide soothing relief.

To use essential oils effectively, perform a patch test on a small area of skin to ensure there are no allergic reactions. Incorporate this topical treatment into your daily routine, especially during flare-ups, and combine it with other management strategies for enhanced results.

Mind-Body Techniques for Holistic Management

Mind-body techniques such as mindfulness, deep breathing, and visualization can significantly impact your overall health and well-being. These practices help manage stress, which is crucial since stress can trigger gout attacks. Incorporating these techniques into your daily routine can enhance your coping mechanisms and reduce symptom severity.

To get started, set aside a few minutes each day for mindfulness exercises or guided meditation sessions.

Many apps and online resources are available to guide beginners. Regular practice can improve your mental resilience and may lead to fewer flare-ups over time.

Exploring Meditation and Yoga for Stress Relief

Meditation and yoga are effective practices for reducing stress and promoting relaxation, which can be beneficial for managing gout. These activities help improve flexibility, reduce tension, and cultivate a sense of calm, potentially lowering the risk of flare-ups. Incorporate gentle yoga poses and meditation techniques into your daily routine.

To practice, start with beginner-level yoga classes or online videos focused on gentle stretching and relaxation. Set aside a dedicated time for meditation, aiming for 5-10 minutes daily to focus on your breath and clear your mind. Regular practice can enhance both physical and emotional well-being.

Dietary Supplements and Their Effectiveness

Dietary supplements, including omega-3 fatty acids and vitamin C, can play a role in gout management by reducing inflammation and supporting joint health. Research suggests that these nutrients may help lower uric acid levels and alleviate symptoms. Incorporating these supplements into your regimen can complement your overall treatment strategy.

To utilize dietary supplements effectively, consult with a healthcare provider to determine the right ones and dosages for your specific situation. Monitor your body's response and discuss any changes in symptoms with your doctor to ensure the supplements are beneficial and safe for you.

Engaging in Gentle Activities Like Tai Chi

Gentle activities like tai chi provide a low-impact way to improve flexibility, balance, and joint function, which can be particularly helpful for those with gout. Practicing tai chi regularly can promote relaxation and reduce stress, which may help prevent flare-ups. Join a local class or follow online tutorials tailored for beginners.

To begin, find a tai chi class that emphasizes gentle movements and proper technique. Practice at home, focusing on slow, deliberate motions, and gradually increase your duration as your comfort level grows. Incorporating tai chi into your routine can foster a holistic approach to managing your condition.

Importance of Research and Evidence-Based Practices

Researching and understanding evidence-based practices is essential for effectively managing gout. Staying informed about the latest findings can help you make educated decisions about your treatment options. Look for reputable sources and peer-reviewed studies to guide your approach to managing symptoms.

Engage in discussions with your healthcare provider about the evidence supporting various treatments, and don't hesitate to ask questions. Being proactive in your research can empower you to take control of your health and ensure that the strategies you choose are grounded in reliable evidence.

CHAPTER 8:

Monitoring and Follow-Up Care

Importance of Regular Medical Check-Ups

Regular medical check-ups are essential for effective gout management. These visits allow healthcare providers to monitor your overall health and specifically assess your uric acid levels, which are crucial for preventing gout flares. During these appointments, your doctor can adjust medications, recommend dietary changes, and identify any complications related to gout.

To make the most of these check-ups, prepare a list of questions and concerns beforehand. This proactive approach ensures that all your health issues are addressed, enabling you to understand better your condition and the steps needed for effective management.

Keeping a Symptom Diary to Track Patterns

Maintaining a symptom diary can significantly aid in managing gout. By recording details about flare-ups, including when they occur, their severity, and any associated activities or foods, you can identify patterns that may trigger your symptoms. This insight is valuable for making informed lifestyle changes and discussing findings with your healthcare provider.

When creating your diary, be consistent in noting symptoms daily. Include specific information like diet, stress levels, and physical activity to help establish a clearer link between your habits and flare-ups, leading to more tailored treatment strategies.

Understanding Lab Tests Related to Gout Management

Lab tests play a critical role in gout management, primarily measuring uric acid levels in the blood. Understanding these tests can help you track your progress and make informed decisions about your treatment. High levels of uric acid can lead to painful gout attacks, so regular monitoring is vital.

To effectively manage gout, familiarize yourself with other tests that may be conducted, such as kidney function tests. Knowing the purpose of each test and discussing results with your doctor will enhance your understanding of your condition and allow you to engage in informed discussions about your treatment options.

Assessing the Effectiveness of Current Treatments

Evaluating the effectiveness of your current treatments is crucial for managing gout. This assessment can involve noting any changes in the frequency and severity of flare-ups, as well as any side effects from medications. By tracking these factors, you can have meaningful discussions with your healthcare provider about potential adjustments.

To assess your treatment's effectiveness, keep a journal detailing your daily symptoms and medication adherence. Regularly review this information with your doctor to ensure that your treatment plan is optimized for your specific needs.

Importance of Open Communication with Healthcare Providers

Open communication with your healthcare provider is fundamental for successful gout management. Sharing your experiences, symptoms, and any concerns can lead to better treatment outcomes. Being honest about medication adherence, lifestyle choices, and how you feel will empower your provider to adjust your plan effectively.

To foster this communication, schedule regular follow-ups and come prepared with questions. Engaging in discussions about your health openly will help you build a strong partnership with your healthcare team, ensuring that you receive personalized care tailored to your situation.

Adjusting Treatment Plans Based on Feedback

Adjusting treatment plans based on feedback is essential for effective gout management. As you monitor your symptoms and communicate with your healthcare provider, you may need to modify medications, dosages, or lifestyle recommendations. This adaptability is crucial for minimizing flare-ups and improving your quality of life.

To facilitate this process, maintain an ongoing dialogue with your healthcare provider. Provide updates on any changes in symptoms or side effects, which can guide necessary adjustments to your treatment plan, ensuring it remains effective over time.

Recognizing Signs of Worsening Conditions

Being able to recognize signs of worsening gout is vital for timely intervention. Symptoms such as increased pain, swelling, or the emergence of new joint pain may indicate that your condition is worsening. Early recognition can help you take action, whether adjusting medications or seeking immediate medical attention.

To stay vigilant, educate yourself on the typical symptoms of gout and their progression. Regular self-assessment and maintaining a symptom diary can help you identify these changes early, allowing for quicker responses to prevent serious complications.

Building a Long-Term Management Plan

Creating a long-term management plan for gout is essential for minimizing flare-ups and maintaining overall health. This plan should include medication adherence, dietary changes, exercise, and regular check-ups. Setting realistic, achievable goals will help you stay committed to your health journey.

When building this plan, involve your healthcare provider to ensure it aligns with your specific needs. Regularly review and adjust your plan as necessary to accommodate any changes in your health status or lifestyle, keeping you on track for long-term success.

Importance of Setting Personal Health Goals

Setting personal health goals is crucial for effectively managing gout. Clear, specific goals can motivate you to make necessary lifestyle changes, such as improving your diet, increasing physical activity, or adhering to medication regimens. These goals provide a sense of direction and achievement as you progress in your health journey.

To set meaningful goals, consider both short-term and long-term objectives. Break larger goals into smaller, manageable steps, and celebrate your achievements along the way. This structured approach will help you stay focused and committed to improving your health.

Incorporating Family Members into Care Strategies

Involving family members in your gout management plan can provide essential support and encouragement. Educating them about your condition allows them to understand your needs and how they can assist, whether by helping with meal prep, reminding you to take medications, or encouraging you to stay active.

To incorporate family members effectively, communicate openly about your condition and treatment plan. Encourage them to participate in healthy activities together, such as cooking nutritious meals or exercising, fostering a supportive environment that contributes to your overall well-being.

Seeking Referrals to Specialists When Needed

If your gout symptoms persist or become complex, seeking referrals to specialists may be necessary. Rheumatologists, for example, have specialized knowledge about gout and can offer advanced treatment options that your primary care provider might not. This step can be crucial in managing more severe or recurring cases.

When seeking a referral, discuss your concerns with your healthcare provider and ask for recommendations based on your specific situation. Don't hesitate to advocate for yourself—getting a second opinion can be beneficial in finding the most effective treatment for your condition.

Staying Informed About New Treatments and Research

Staying informed about new treatments and research related to gout can empower you to make better health decisions. Advances in medication, dietary recommendations, and management strategies are continually evolving. Being aware of these developments can lead to more effective management of your condition.

To keep up-to-date, follow reputable health organizations, read medical journals, or join support groups where new information is shared. Engaging with communities can also provide emotional support and practical tips from others experiencing similar challenges.

Utilizing Technology for Health Monitoring (Apps)

Utilizing technology, such as health monitoring apps, can greatly enhance your gout management strategy. These apps can help you track symptoms, medication adherence, and dietary habits, providing valuable data to share with your healthcare provider. Many apps also offer reminders for medication and appointments.

To effectively use these tools, choose an app that aligns with your specific needs and preferences. Regularly input your data and review the trends it reveals, which can facilitate informed discussions with your doctor, leading to improved management of your gout condition.

CHAPTER 9:

Common Concerns and FAQs

Can Gout Affect More Than One Joint at a Time?

Yes, gout can affect multiple joints simultaneously, particularly during a flare-up. This condition often starts in one joint, most commonly the big toe, but as it progresses, it can impact other joints like the ankles, knees, and fingers. When gout attacks several joints, it can lead to increased pain and swelling, making mobility difficult.

To manage multi-joint gout, it's essential to consult with a healthcare provider. They may recommend anti-inflammatory medications to reduce pain and swelling, as well as lifestyle changes that focus on diet and exercise to help prevent future attacks.

What Are the Long-Term Effects of Untreated Gout?

Untreated gout can lead to serious long-term complications, such as chronic joint damage and the formation of tophi, which are large deposits of uric acid crystals that can develop under the skin. These deposits may lead to deformities and persistent pain, severely impacting quality of life.

Additionally, untreated gout increases the risk of kidney stones and kidney disease, as excess uric acid can accumulate in the kidneys. Regular check-ups and blood tests can help monitor uric acid levels, guiding effective treatment and minimizing long-term complications.

How Can I Prevent Gout Attacks from Recurring?

Preventing recurring gout attacks involves a combination of medication, lifestyle changes, and dietary adjustments. Regularly taking medications prescribed by your doctor, such as allopurinol, can help maintain lower uric acid levels. It's also essential to stay hydrated by drinking plenty of water, as this can help flush out uric acid.

Incorporating a balanced diet low in purines—found in red meat, organ meats, and seafood—can significantly reduce the likelihood of flare-ups. Regular physical activity, maintaining a healthy weight, and avoiding high-fructose beverages can also help manage uric acid levels and prevent attacks.

Is Gout Hereditary?

Yes, gout can be hereditary. If you have a family history of gout, you may be at a higher risk of developing the condition due to genetic factors that affect how your body processes uric acid. Understanding your family history can help you take preventive measures early.

To mitigate hereditary risks, maintaining a healthy lifestyle is crucial. Regular check-ups and discussions with your doctor about your family history can also help you monitor uric acid levels and manage your risk effectively.

Can Diet Alone Control Gout?

While diet plays a significant role in managing gout, it is usually not enough to control the condition by itself. A diet low in purines can help reduce uric acid levels, but it should be combined with medication and lifestyle changes for optimal management. Foods rich in whole grains, fruits, and vegetables can aid in lowering uric acid.

To effectively use diet as part of your management strategy, consider consulting a dietitian who specializes in gout. They can help you create a personalized meal plan that includes foods that help reduce uric acid and identifies those to limit or avoid.

What Should I Do During a Gout Flare-Up?

During a gout flare-up, the first step is to rest the affected joint and elevate it to reduce swelling. Applying ice packs for 15-20 minutes can help alleviate pain and inflammation. Over-the-counter anti-inflammatory medications like ibuprofen can also be effective, but consult your doctor before taking any medication.

It's important to stay hydrated during a flare-up, as fluids can help flush uric acid from your system. If pain persists or worsens, seek medical advice for potential prescription medications that can provide stronger relief.

Are There Specific Foods I Should Avoid Completely?

Yes, certain foods are high in purines and should be avoided or limited if you have gout. These include red meats, organ meats (like liver), certain seafood (such as sardines and anchovies), and sugary drinks containing high fructose corn syrup. Alcohol, particularly beer, can also trigger gout attacks and should be consumed with caution.

To maintain a healthy diet, focus on consuming low-purine options such as low-fat dairy, whole grains, fruits, and vegetables. Keeping a food diary can help you track your meals and identify any food triggers related to your gout.

How Does Weight Loss Impact Gout Management?

Weight loss can have a positive effect on gout management by reducing uric acid levels and the frequency of attacks. Excess body weight increases the production of uric acid and can hinder its elimination, leading to higher risk for gout. Gradual weight loss through a balanced diet and exercise can help lower uric acid levels effectively.

To achieve weight loss goals, aim for a healthy, sustainable plan that includes regular physical activity and portion control. Consulting a healthcare professional or a registered dietitian can provide guidance on creating a tailored plan that suits your lifestyle.

What Role Does Exercise Play in Managing Gout?

Regular exercise plays a vital role in managing gout by helping maintain a healthy weight and improving overall joint function. Low-impact activities such as walking, swimming, or cycling can enhance circulation and flexibility without putting undue stress on the joints.

Incorporating strength training can also be beneficial for overall health. Aim for at least 150 minutes of moderate exercise per week, and consider consulting a fitness professional to develop a suitable exercise regimen tailored to your needs and limitations.

Are There Any Specific Supplements Recommended?

Certain supplements may help manage gout symptoms, though you should always consult a healthcare provider before starting any new regimen. Cherry extract and vitamin C have been shown in some studies to potentially lower uric acid levels and reduce the frequency of gout attacks.

Omega-3 fatty acids, commonly found in fish oil, may also help reduce inflammation associated with gout. A healthcare professional can guide you in selecting appropriate supplements and dosages based on your individual health needs.

Can I Still Drink Alcohol If I Have Gout?

While it's not necessary to eliminate alcohol completely, moderation is key for those with gout. Beer and spirits are known to trigger gout attacks, while moderate consumption of wine may have a lesser impact. It's advisable to limit alcohol intake and observe how your body responds.

If you choose to drink, stay hydrated by alternating alcoholic beverages with water. Monitoring your uric acid levels and discussing alcohol consumption with your healthcare provider can help you understand your personal limits.

What Is the Relationship Between Gout and Other Health Conditions?

Gout is often associated with other health conditions, including hypertension, diabetes, and kidney disease. Elevated uric acid levels can contribute to these conditions, making it essential to manage gout effectively to reduce the risk of complications.

Regular medical check-ups can help identify any coexisting health issues. It's important to communicate with your healthcare provider about all your health concerns to create a comprehensive management plan that addresses gout and any related conditions.

When Should I Seek Immediate Medical Attention for Gout?

Immediate medical attention is warranted if you experience severe pain, swelling, or redness in your joints that does not improve with at-home care. Additionally, if you develop a fever or notice any signs of infection, such as pus or increased warmth around the joint, seek medical help promptly.

If you have frequent flare-ups or your current treatment plan is not effective, it's also crucial to consult with your healthcare provider for possible adjustments. Early intervention can help prevent complications and improve overall management of your condition.

Conclusion:

Recap of the Importance of Understanding Gout Triggers

Understanding gout triggers is crucial for effective management and prevention of flare-ups. Gout is often triggered by high levels of uric acid in the blood, which can accumulate in joints, leading to intense pain and inflammation. Identifying personal triggers—such as specific foods, medications, or lifestyle factors—can empower individuals to make informed choices and avoid situations that might provoke a gout attack.

Keeping a food diary or tracking symptoms can help pinpoint these triggers more accurately.

Moreover, recognizing how triggers interact with one another can provide deeper insights into managing this condition. For example, combining certain foods or excessive alcohol consumption with dehydration can increase uric acid levels. By maintaining awareness and understanding these triggers, individuals can proactively take steps to reduce their risk of future attacks.

Emphasis on the Role of Lifestyle Changes in Prevention

Lifestyle changes play a pivotal role in preventing gout flare-ups and managing overall health. A diet low in purines—found in red meats, organ meats, and some seafood—can significantly decrease uric acid levels. Instead, individuals should focus on incorporating more fruits, vegetables, whole grains, and low-fat dairy into their meals. Staying hydrated by drinking plenty of water also helps the body excrete uric acid more efficiently.

Additionally, regular physical activity can assist in maintaining a healthy weight, which is essential since obesity is a major risk factor for gout. Simple changes, like walking regularly or incorporating strength training into your routine, can lead to significant improvements in overall health and uric acid management.

Encouragement to Consult Healthcare Professionals for Personalized Plans

Consulting healthcare professionals is essential for developing a personalized gout management plan. Doctors can provide comprehensive assessments that take into account individual health history, symptoms, and lifestyle factors. This tailored approach allows for the identification of the most effective treatment options, including medication, dietary recommendations, and lifestyle changes that suit personal circumstances.

Healthcare professionals can also guide the proper use of medications to lower uric acid levels and manage pain during flare-ups. Regular follow-ups can ensure that the management plan is effective and can be adjusted as needed. Building a strong relationship with a healthcare provider fosters a supportive environment for managing gout effectively.

Importance of Ongoing Education and Support in Managing Gout

Ongoing education about gout is vital for successful management. Knowledge of the condition, including its symptoms, causes, and treatment options, enables individuals to make informed decisions about their health. Resources such as support groups, educational workshops, and reputable online materials can enhance understanding and provide valuable insights into living with gout.

Furthermore, surrounding oneself with supportive family and friends can play a significant role in managing gout. Encouragement from loved ones can help individuals adhere to lifestyle changes and treatment plans. Sharing experiences within support groups can also offer practical tips and foster a sense of community.

Maintaining a positive outlook is fundamental to effectively managing gout. Stress can trigger flare-ups, so incorporating relaxation techniques—such as mindfulness, meditation, or yoga—can be beneficial. A proactive mindset encourages individuals to take control of their health by implementing necessary changes, monitoring triggers, and seeking support when needed.

Adopting a proactive approach also involves regular check-ups and open communication with healthcare providers. By staying informed and engaged in their own care, individuals can better manage their condition and enhance their quality of life. Emphasizing positivity and resilience can transform the journey of living with gout into one of empowerment and growth.

www.ingramcontent.com/pod-product-compliance
Lightning Source LLC
Chambersburg PA
CBHW071029250726
48653CB00005B/1771